Holistic Health:

Natural
Liver
Detox

I0441697

An All-Natural Way to Restore Optimal Liver Functioning

RON KNESS

Published by:

Ron Kness Writing and Publishing

Gold Canyon, AZ

United States of America

ISBN-13: 978-1535259323

ISBN-10: 1535259329

Contents

Disclaimer

This publication is for informational purposes only and is not intended as medical advice. Medical advice should always be obtained from a qualified medical professional for any health conditions or symptoms associated with them.

Every possible effort has been made in preparing and researching this material. We make no warranties with respect to the accuracy, applicability of its contents or any omissions.

Introduction

We live in a world that is chockfull of toxins be it in the air we breathe, our food, our water... so much so that their entrance into our bodies has become unavoidable.

Exposure to these toxins requires that all of the organs in your body work in synergy to maintain homeostasis - meaning everything needs to be in a certain balance in order to function optimally. If the function of one organ or system goes awry, the others will also be affected.

Your liver and kidneys play a vital role of filtering toxins out of your body, but your liver has an additional function of breaking down the present toxins in order to expel them from your body.

This enzymatic process occurs in two phases – breaking down the toxins and bonding these broken parts to other molecules that destroy the toxic substances and expel them from your body through sweat, urine and fecal matter.

When the liver becomes overburdened or overworked due to chronic exposure to toxins via the environment, diet, smoking, alcohol use, lack of sleep or poor stress management, it can slow down and cause a back-up of toxins in your system. This can impact many other systems and organs in your body resulting in various symptoms.

The following are just a few common symptoms of an improperly functioning liver:

- Weight gain/difficulty losing weight

- Fluid buildup in the belly or abdomen

- Bruise easily

- Painful gallstones

- Chronic itching

- Yellowing of the skin and eyes (jaundice)

- Kidney failure

- Muscle loss

- Loss of appetite

- Unsightly skin conditions and liver spots

- Spider-like veins in the skin

- Low energy and frequent weakness (fatigue)

- Mental confusion as toxins build up in the blood

- A weakened immune system, leaving you unguarded against sickness, disease and infection

After reading the many potential consequences of a toxic liver, you may be wondering how you can support your liver to make sure it is functioning at its optimal level.

Many people think that by just making a few tweaks to their diet they can counteract the effects of toxic buildup. It is true that following a nutrient dense diet will support your liver and can help however, it doesn't have the same impact as cleansing/detoxing.

A cleansing program takes it a step further by helping eliminate the stored toxins therefore allowing your liver to reboot and rejuvenate.

Benefits of a Liver Detox

You experience any of the problems mentioned earlier, then you should suspect that your liver may need some special attention. Ignoring these signs will only make things worse and could put you at risk for developing a host of other minor and major health problems.

Rather than ignore your symptoms, be proactive and take control of your health by committing to a program that can help to restore and rejuvenate your body.

One of the simplest and most effective ways to reboot and rejuvenate your liver is to do a natural liver detox or cleansing.

Liver detoxification is basically a program that is designed to purge your liver of the toxins and other harmful particles that impede it from functioning properly. This is best done naturally through the use of various superfoods and supplements that have a direct, positive impact on the liver.

Be aware of any detox program that advises you to consume only liquids and/or severely restrict calories. Liquid fasts can be dangerous and should only be done under the care of a medical professional.

The liver needs much more than liquids to heal - adequate amounts of lean protein, fiber and other nutrients are necessary in order to for it to thrive so it is essential that these are present in any liver detox meal plan.

It is not necessary to go to extremes to cleanse your liver – a healthy, well planned diet and some positive lifestyle tweaks are enough to see amazing results.

There are many incredible benefits of a liver detox. Below are just a few of the health advantages you get when you follow a proven liver detox program.

Weight loss: A liver detox improves your body's ability to produce bile so that it can effectively burn out fats from within the body. This results in weight loss by improving the metabolism of fats. *(Many who undergo a liver detox mention achieving weight loss that had eluded them for years, even though they tried every diet program under the sun.)*

A strong, healthy immune system: A liver detox improves the liver's capacity to remove toxins and other poisons from your body. This means restoring your body's natural defense system, so *you fight infection, disease, inflammation and sickness effortlessly.*

Prevents formation of painful liver stones: Liver stones are caused by the hardening of bile into small stones. This condition arises from having too much cholesterol in the body. The liver stones can block the gallbladder and liver. This prevents both organs from functioning properly. Doing a liver detox helps purge the liver of these tiny and painful stones.

Supports natural, holistic detox: The liver detox does not only cleanse the liver from harmful substances. It also supports holistic body detoxification.

A holistic approach means understanding that your physical and mental health are connected, as are all physical body parts and body processes.

This means once you start doing a liver detox you also help the other organs of your body, *positively affecting and improving health inside and out from head to toe, both mentally and physically.*

Improves energy: Toxic buildup in the bloodstream can result in a constant lack of energy, and feeling of weakness. *A natural liver detox returns your vigor and vitality, rewarding you with naturally high energy levels.*

These are not the energetic spikes and crashes provided by sugar and unhealthy food. Instead, you can count on healthy, natural energy to easily get through your daily routine, without resorting to sugar, caffeine and other less than healthy energy boosters.

Improves your "glow": Undergoing a liver detox restores the glow and vitality of your body. Have you ever heard someone refer to another person as "glowing"? Others will be saying this about you, and you will notice it yourself. Your improved level of health and vitality is manifested in the quality and appearance of your skin and hair. *You can take off years off your physical appearance with a simple liver detox.*

Incredible anti-aging properties: You can look and feel 5 to 20 years younger simply by undergoing a natural liver detox.

This is because all of your bodily processes depend on a healthy functioning liver to rid your body of poison toxins and waste. You will literally look and feel younger, healthier and stronger, improve your brain function and energy levels, all from a simple and natural liver detox.

Who Needs a Liver Detox?

Quite frankly, not everyone needs a liver detox or cleansing. If you eat a perfect diet on a fairly regular basis…lots of healthy fruits and vegetables, whole grains, nuts and seeds, and very little processed or fast foods, your liver may be in great shape. In this case, a detox program is probably not necessary.

The plain truth of the matter, however, is that the average person does not always put the right types of foods and beverages into his or her body these days.

Another scary realization is that even if you enjoy a wonderfully healthy diet, exercise frequently, drink lots of water and get sufficient sleep, the poisons and toxins in the air you breathe can still keep your liver from functioning properly.

This is why a liver detox is becoming a popular option for people who are looking for holistic approaches to improving their health.

You simply monitor and change the things you put into your body, and your internal processes reward you with wonderful health from head to toe.

So, who needs a liver detox? Should it only be limited to people with an unhealthy or toxic liver or is it a smart move for everyone? Below are the kinds of people who will benefit from a liver detox.

Men and women who are overweight or obese:
Overweight and obese individuals are at a higher risk for developing Type 2 diabetes. They also suffer more cardiovascular, circulatory and respiratory problems than those who are not overweight or obese. How many people are either overweight or obese today?

The National Health and Nutrition Examination Survey of 2010 revealed that 68% of adults in modern countries are either overweight or obese. That means in a group of 100 people, 68 could lose unhealthy body fat and weight by participating in an easy-to-follow, natural liver detox. Even if you're not overweight, a liver detox can help you shed a few pounds naturally.

Stressed individuals: Stress can be an indication of an overworked and poorly functioning liver. Moreover, stressed people tend to have unhealthy lifestyle habits such as eating fatty foods and drinking alcohol. *If you suffer from frequent stress, anxiety and depression, a liver detox may provide the calming peace of mind you have been looking for.*

People in their 40s: If you are already in your 40s, chances are that you might be feeling some changes in your body. This means your energy level is not as high as before. You may notice changes in your skin and hair that definitely don't make you smile. *Even if you have lived a fairly healthy lifestyle you still cannot escape the fact that your body has accumulated a lot of toxins over the years.*

Doing a liver detox can help return your liver to a healthy state, so you enjoy healthy body weight regulation, young and strong looking and feeling hair and skin, "all day" energy and the other benefits a natural liver detox offers.

Anyone suffering from the following conditions: Fatigue, brain fog, chronic joint or muscle pain, migraines, digestive problems, insomnia, autoimmune disease, hormonal imbalance, acne, skin rashes, depression, allergies, chronic bad breath, chemical sensitivity and rapid weight gain.

Remember, your liver powers many bodily processes. So health symptoms you may not connect to an unhealthy liver can be effectively treated with a liver detox. A healthy, properly functioning liver can reverse the above conditions, and many more.

How Your Liver Works

The liver is the largest gland organ in the human body. It secretes a fluid called bile which is necessary for digesting fats so that they can be easily absorbed by the intestine. It has an average weight of 3 pounds and is located in the upper right area of the abdomen, just underneath the diaphragm and to the right of the stomach. It receives 1.5 quarts of blood every minute through the portal vein and hepatic artery.

Within the liver are tiny cells called hepatocytes which are mainly responsible for the hundreds of functions of this gland in the body. Aside from producing bile for fat breakdown, below are the functions of a robust liver in maintaining a healthy human body.

Carbohydrate synthesis: The liver plays a vital role in the metabolic synthesis of carbohydrates. A well-functioning liver can synthesize 100 grams of glycogen through the process of glycogenesis for carbohydrate metabolism. It is also responsible for the production of glycerol which is necessary for the synthesis of glucose by breaking down fat cells.

Protein metabolism: The liver is also responsible for the metabolism of protein. It produces clotting factors like the fibrinogen, prothrombin, and anti-thrombin. It is also the main site for the red blood cell production of fetuses.

Lipid metabolism: The liver produces bile that breaks down cholesterol through the process of lipogenesis.

It is also involved in the production of triglycerides as well as other lipoproteins.

Storage: It stores different substances such as glycogen, Vitamin D, A, K, and B12. It stores iron and copper as well.

Detoxifies blood: The liver also helps rid harmful substances in the blood such as drugs and alcohol. When we drink alcohol, eat a poor diet full of processed and fast foods, or take a lot of medicines, our liver is working non-stop to detoxify our blood from the harmful substances. The liver filter can also remove a wide variety of contaminants like fungi, bacteria, virus and parasites in the bloodstream so they don't build up in the blood and cause health problems.

Destroys old red blood cells: Old red blood cells go to the liver to get destroyed and eliminated through the digestive system as waste. The liver cells are separated by spaces that act as a filter. Blood flows through the filter, which removes old blood cells, chemicals, drugs as well as other harmful substances from the body. This filter is called the sinusoidal system and is carried out by specialized cells called Kupffer cells which have the ability to break down toxic substances.

Produces angiotensinogen: Angiotensinogen is a hormone that raises the blood pressure once activated by an enzyme called renin, which is released by the kidney. If the liver is not functioning well, elevated blood pressure may be experienced.

Produces albumin: Albumin is a protein found in the blood serum and it is important in maintaining the oncotic pressure and transporting of the steroid hormones and fatty acids.

Remove chemical toxins: There are more than 1,000 toxins that are found in the food, water, and even air that we take in. All of these can cause harm to our body. Our liver is one of our first lines of defenses and it renders these chemicals inert by breaking them down and turning them into waste that is eliminated as urine or feces.

The liver contributes to a lot of functions within the body, so it is important to maintain the healthy state of homeostasis. Unfortunately, many people suffer from liver diseases over time due to their lifestyle and habits.

This is why it is so important to have a natural, drug-free, liver detox regularly so you give your liver a break. (Especially if you eat processed and fast foods on a regular basis.)

Symptoms of a Toxic Liver

Y ou are probably asking yourself, "How do I know if my liver is toxic?" It is not always easy to determine if a liver is functioning poorly. The reason is that there are many conditions that are associated with a sick liver that arise from different causes. Symptoms like irritability and fatigue may indicate a toxic liver but they can also be caused by a multitude of factors.

A doctor may tell you your chronic fatigue arises from stress and a poor diet. Those problems may actually be contributing to a poorly functioning liver, but because toxic liver symptoms are so common to other conditions, you are diagnosed incorrectly.

Once you experience multiple adverse health conditions regularly, this could be a sign that you have an unhealthy liver. Remember that the liver's main function is to rid the body of harmful substances. So if it is not working properly, a long list of negative health conditions and symptoms can arise.

How do you know if your liver is not functioning well? Below are the symptoms of a toxic liver.

Superficial symptoms

Superficial symptoms refer to signs that you can see on your body. This means you can simply step up to a mirror, or look at your body and identify symptoms.

These involve the color of your eyes, skin or even the condition of your mouth. Below are the superficial symptoms that possibly indicate a problematic liver.

Eyes: Having a toxic liver can be manifested through the eyes. As the windows to our souls, we can tell that something is wrong in our internal body through the condition of our eyes. For instance, if you experience chronic itching, redness or puffiness in your eyes and you are not allergic to anything, it can indicate a problem in your liver. Take note of the color of your eyes. If you see a yellow tinge on the whites of your eyes, it can be an indication of jaundice, which is a sign of a toxic and severely damaged liver.

Skin: The skin can tell if the liver is functioning well or not. (This needs to be repeated, because it is so important. If you have chronic skin conditions of any sort, this could be a sign of a poorly functioning liver. This is one of the easiest and earliest toxic liver symptoms to spot.) If you feel itchy at all times or mysterious brown spots or blemishes appear on your skin, then you can suspect something is wrong with your liver.

Other signs you need to look for include a yellowish hue on the skin, rashes such as eczema, extreme acne breakouts and the emergence of gross body odor. The visible appearance of blood vessels on the face can also indicate a problem, as well as the itchiness of your palms and the soles of your feet.

A toxic liver can also be manifested through bad breath and a coated tongue. However, such symptoms are often mistaken for other diseases thus it is important to look for the major signs and symptoms of a toxic liver.

Major Symptoms

While the superficial symptoms are not always reliable in identifying the presence of liver disease, looking at the major symptoms can help you confirm that your liver is suffering severely. Below are the major signs that identify a toxic liver.

(If you have more than one of the following major symptoms, and one or more of the minor or superficial symptoms, you should take some kind of treatment action as soon as possible. A natural liver detox can be implemented immediately, and goes to work instantly returning your liver to its naturally healthy state. However, it is important to always consult with a physician regarding your symptoms and discuss your plans to try a natural approach to improving your health.)

Poor immunity: Since the liver is mainly responsible for removing contaminants and toxic substance from the body, a damaged liver often results to having a low immune system. This means you find yourself falling prey to sickness, infections, colds and flus frequently.

A person with a toxic liver often experiences inflammation, fibromyalgia, chronic fatigue syndrome and recurring infections. Autoimmune diseases may also arise from having a poor liver. These conditions indicate a weakening of your body's natural defense systems.

Blood sugar problems: Type 2 diabetes may also be associated with a toxic liver. In fact, it is one of the symptoms of a fatty liver disease. Remember that one of the functions of the liver is the storage of glucose.

A fatty liver disease means your liver is incapable of removing glucose from the blood. So if you suffer from Type 2 diabetes, then you should suspect a toxic liver.

Impaired cognition and brain function: The liver is often referred to as the seat of anger because you often feel angry and agitated if it is not functioning well. This has something to do with the inability of a damaged liver to detoxify the body from harmful substances. Once these (harmful substances) build up in the bloodstream, it affects all of your other organs as well.

As a result, having a toxic liver causes distress particularly to the nervous system. This means chronic headaches occur, as well as heightened levels of anxiety, stress, depression, impaired cognition, and drastic mood changes.

Digestive problems: Bile is produced in the liver to aid in digestion. A toxic liver wreaks havoc on the digestive system which can lead to problems like indigestion, constipation, irritable bowel syndrome, acid reflux, vomiting, and hemorrhoids. Gallstones may also result from a poorly functioning liver, as well as intolerance to alcohol and fatty foods. This is often manifested by bloating.

Slow metabolism: A slow metabolism means weight gain. Your metabolic process is how efficiently you burn calories. When your liver is not functioning well, your metabolism slows down to a snail's pace so you likely gain weight easily. Having a roll of fat tissues in the abdominal area is an indication that the liver is not functioning properly.

This happens because the liver does not produce enough bile to break down fats and remove it as wastes. As a result, fat easily builds around the organs as visceral fats, which can lead to elevated cholesterol levels and an increased risk of cardiovascular diseases.

(If you have tried in vain to lose weight and burn body fat, it may not be your fault. It is not a cause of laziness or lack of willpower. It may just be that you need a healthy liver detox to lose the extra body weight which has been frustrating you for so many years.)

Once you suspect yourself of having a toxic liver, you can confirm your condition by undergoing a liver-function test. If you determine your liver is toxic, and is not functioning properly, a natural liver detox is your first step to looking and feeling healthy once again.

Simple Steps to a Healthier Liver

G oogle "liver detox" and you will find millions of results. There are a lot of liver detox programs out there. The ones that are effective for creating optimal health all have one thing in common …

They include dietary changes and supplements to cleanse your liver, return it to its naturally functioning state, and keep your liver working properly in the future.

Eating the right foods and supplements can quickly create a healthy, strong liver that does its job properly. As part of a smart liver detox, as well as practices that are part of a healthy lifestyle, do the following:

Drink lots of water: The Mayo Clinic, American Cancer Foundation, WebMD, Arthritis Foundation and other respected health authorities offer the same advice regarding water consumption - ***you should be ingesting a minimum of 1 gallon (3.8 litres) of water each and every day.***

This includes not only water that you drink, but water that is naturally found in the foods that you eat. Drinking water helps the kidneys flush out toxins and poisons. Your kidneys and liver work together to cleanse your body, thus drinking water can help improve the detoxification of both organs.

Avoid supplements containing iron: Iron supplements can damage the liver over time. A person who takes iron supplements may have iron overload that can cause damage to the liver cells, eventually leading to their deaths. This results in scarring which can lead to liver cirrhosis.

It also increases the probability that the DNA of your cells is damaged and changed, and increases the risk of developing cancer of the liver.

Eat a lot of high fiber fruits and vegetables: Fruits and vegetables that contain a lot of fiber prevent the liver from overworking. The fiber slows down the absorption of glucose by the liver so it does not overwork the organ too much. A high fiber diet has also been linked to a healthy body weight regulation.

Split peas, beans, artichokes and broccoli are extremely high in healthy dietary fiber. So are Brussels sprouts, raspberries, blackberries and other berries, avocados and pears.

Glutathione: Glutathione is an important antioxidant produced naturally by the body. It is made up of three amino acids – glutamine, glycine, and cysteine. It traps free radicals as well as toxins such as mercury and other heavy metals so they get flushed out. Aside from being naturally produced by the body, glutathione can also be obtained by eating certain fruits and vegetables.

Squash, zucchini, potatoes and melons deliver healthy glutathione. Garlic, spinach, asparagus, grapefruit, strawberries and peaches also contain this liver-friendly compound.

Avoid animal products: Animal products may contain a lot of substances like antibiotics, hormones, and steroids. Moreover, they also contain saturated fats that can elevate the amount of cholesterol in the body which can impede the detoxification process of the liver.

Exercise: Do not underestimate the power of exercise. Adding heat to the body through exercise helps mobilize the toxins out of the fat and muscle cells so that they are eliminated as sweat. Be sure to engage in an activity that feels good to you and is something you enjoy. Yoga, walking, stretching, hiking, biking, rebounding (jumping on a trampoline) and swimming are all great ways to get started.

Sauna: Using a sauna can be a great addition to your detox strategy. There are numerous benefits including the elimination of toxins.

Lemon Water – Starting your day with a glass of warm lemon water is a gentle yet effective way to support and cleanse the liver, kidneys, and colon, and will help to alkalize the body. It will assist in breaking up mucus and will provide energy via enzymes, vitamin C, potassium, and trace minerals. First thing in the morning, before breakfast squeeze the juice from half of a fresh lemon (do not use bottled varieties) and mix with 8oz of warm water.

Toxin Elimination Bath – Epsom salts have a myriad of benefits including reducing pain and inflammation and infusing your body with magnesium. Magnesium is an essential nutrient that plays a vital role in your overall health including the elimination of toxins. Most people are deficient in this nutrient and therefore taking an Epsom salt bath should be an important part of your detox strategy. Each evening, place 2 cups of Epsom salts under running water at the hottest level you can tolerate. You can also add essential oils such as lavender oil for a destressing aromatherapy effect. Soak for at least 20 to 30 minutes and allow yourself to sweat. You should feel very relaxed and sleep soundly.

Fiber – Fiber is an essential component to your liver detox because it helps to support the colon in its role of toxin elimination. In addition to lots of fresh vegetables, ground flax seeds and chia seeds are recommended.

Body Brushing – The lymphatic system plays an important role in detoxing your body and body brushing (or dry brushing) is an effective way to stimulate the lymph nodes in keeping blood and other vital tissues detoxified. The many benefits include breaking up cellulite, removing dead skin, promoting circulation, and strengthening your immune system. You will need to use a natural bristle brush, which can be purchased at most health food stores or pharmacies. The entire process should take approximately 2-3 minutes and should be done prior to showering or your taking your detox bath. Start at your feet and work up the body in long strokes towards your heart. Be sure to cover the whole body, but skip the face and the breasts.

Castor oil packs – These packs can have a very profound impact on the health of your liver – despite that they are an external method of detoxing.

Castor oil has been found to have anti-inflammatory effects when used externally. You can apply the oil to your skin (stomach area) via a pack and it can be used to stimulate and detox the liver and gall bladder.

Directions:

- You will need 100% pure, cold-pressed castor oil, a piece of cloth (wool flannel is said to be best), and a hot water bottle (or heating pad). If you don't want to go searching for the supplies, you can purchase a castor oil pack online.

- Fold the cloth into three or four layers, and soak it with castor oil.

- Rub castor oil on your stomach, lie down, and place the hot flannel on top of your stomach.

- Seal off the flannel with plastic wrap.

- Cover with a hot water bottle or heating pad for one hour, keeping the flannel as hot as safely and comfortably possible.

- After you are done, wash the oil from your abdomen then relax. Many people report a very serene and tranquil feeling after completing this detox regimen.

Although it is regarded as a safe regimen you must always consult your doctor before trying any new program or alternative remedy.

Foods to Eat for a Healthy Liver

Many people don't believe that illness can be prevented through eating healthy because it just seems too simple or even quirky. We have been led to believe that you have little control over whether or not you develop an illness because it's already pre-programmed in your DNA.

While this may be true for some types of ailments, it is not so for all. There is tremendous power in nutrition and what you put into our body can make a major difference in whether or not you develop certain illnesses.

There are countless superfoods that can prevent, manage and possibly even reverse some diseases. Below, we've curated a list of the top 20 superfoods that have the power to ward off toxins, reduce inflammation, reset your metabolism, nurture your skin and most importantly, heal your body.

The Perils of a Toxic Diet

A toxic diet made up of sugars, starches, sodium, additives, preservatives and other negative ingredients can do more harm than just weight gain. Of course obesity is one truly negative factor, but toxic diets also cause inflammation of organs and internal structures and debilitating and potentially deadly diseases such as heart disease and diabetes.

Aside from disease and weight gain, toxic diets also lead to decreased energy levels, lack of motivation and laziness, insomnia and irregular sleeping patterns, depression and anxiety, chronic fatigue, mental fogginess, and increased stress. A toxic diet can truly hold you back from enjoying life to its fullest and embracing the positive.

Superfoods to the Rescue

Not only do superfoods boost body and mind power but they will work to open up new channels of positivity and tranquility in your life.

These simple, natural, and healthy staples provide health and life benefits such as:
- Increased metabolism
- Reduced inflammation
- Healthy, glowing skin
- Reduced cravings for junk foods
- Better sleeping habits
- Improved cognitive function
- Weight loss
- Increased energy
- Improved mood

Contrary to what many think, superfoods do not have to be expensive, hard to find, or complicated. These simple, healthy, and effective foods can help you break the chains of your toxic diet and achieve heightened health, positive thinking, and an elevated enjoyment of life.

20 Superfoods to Heal Your Body

There is a plethora of information out there on superfoods, so it can be confusing to know where to start. Here is a list of the top 20 superfoods that will work to heal your body from the damages of a toxic diet and put you on the path to a healthier and happier lifestyle.

Blackberries

When it comes to improving your immune system, blackberries are incredibly effective due to their rich nutrient content. With their extremely high vitamin C and vitamin K levels, blackberries speed up wound recovery, strengthen tissues, and regulate blood clotting. Low in carbs and fats but very high in protein, blackberries are definitely among the most nutritious foods out there, not to mention the tastiest. As a simple snack, all you have to do is wash them off and eat away. A half cup will give you all the benefits you need.

Cranberries

Speaking of vitamins C and K, cranberries are also packed full of these effective and helpful vitamins. These delicious red berries do more than just boost your immune system. Their components work as a powerful antioxidant and anti-inflammatory, plus contain many essential anti-cancer properties. A half cup of these delicious fruits will go a long way toward giving you the nutrients your body deserves.

Raspberries

With raspberries you have a powerful antioxidant due to their being full of vitamin C and ellagic acid. These berries also boast a high amount of anti-inflammatory properties, making them an important part of any superfood diet. Like with the other berries on this list, a half cup will be sufficient to give you these benefits and will also serve as a very tasty snack.

Blueberries

Blueberries are known as an antioxidant superfood that not only has vitamin C, but is high in potassium and even phytoflavinoids. Eating blueberries daily has been shown to have a dramatic effect on your skin by helping to reduce lines and wrinkles. Research suggests they also reduce a type of cardiovascular disease and even ward off cancer. It's recommended that ½ to 1 cup is eaten every day for its full benefits. Note: Cultivated blueberries are the typical ones you buy in the grocery store. Whenever possible, buy wild blueberries (usually found in the frozen food section). They have double the antioxidant power as cultivated.

Limes

Limes are beneficial for more than just adding flavor to various foods and drinks. The same flavonoids that give limes their unique flavor also provide a wide range of antioxidant and anti-cancer benefits, plus combat free radicals. Limes are also packed full of vitamin C. Since limes are very sour, just one lime will do for a serving. Even with just one per week you will receive incredible benefits, making limes one of the top superfoods on this list.

Black Beans

When it comes to providing a plethora of benefits, black beans really stand out. Containing both phosphorous and iron, black beans help maintain bone structure and maintain the strength and elasticity of the bones as well. The protein contained in these beans makes for healthy mucous membranes and vitamin B1 aids the body in breaking down fat. Needless to say, a quarter cup of black beans will do your body right.

Rhubarb

You may not think of rhubarb as being in anything other than pies, but its ultra-high vitamin K level puts it firmly in the superfood category. Vitamin K plays a major role in brain health and also greatly aids neuronal health. Plus, at just 11 calories per serving, rhubarb distinguishes itself as a healthy and incredibly effective superfood.

Kidney Beans

When it comes to kidney beans, the main beneficial aspects are their frolic acid and their phosphorus. With the phosphorous being vital for cellular regulation and the frolic acid providing help in preventing cancer-causing DNA mutations and also assisting in cellular health, kidney beans come packed with many benefits. With just a half cup serving, your body will absorb multiple benefits.

Edamame

Edamame comes packed with folic acid and vitamin K, giving consumers valuable assistance with brain health and nervous system maintenance. These beans also help the body produce new cells, which greatly combat the effects of aging. In just a half cup serving, edamame really packs on the health benefits.

Navy Beans

These tasty and useful beans are full of a very vital component which pushes them into the top tier of superfoods. Vitamin B1 works to help your body convert blood sugar into pure energy, providing consumers a natural and healthy energy source. It also works to keep the mucous membranes healthy, which is essential for proper nervous system function. Just a half cup of navy beans will put you on the path to nervous system health and provide a needed dose of natural energy.

Lentils

Just like with navy beans, lentils have the vitamin B1 that will aid your body in converting blood sugar into energy. Another aspect that really puts lentils at the top of the superfoods chain is their high level of lean protein. A quarter cup of lentils in the recipe of your choice will give you an extra boost of energy as well as a dose of healthy protein that will allow your body to function at a truly high level.

Asparagus Spears

Asparagus is full of essentials such as vitamin K and folic acid, providing the bodily benefits connected to each. What really sets asparagus apart from the other superfoods on this list is the addition of chromium. This trace mineral works to enhance insulin's ability to transport glucose to the cells from the bloodstream. In addition, asparagus brings another essential to the table: fiber. Fiber greatly aids digestion and the body's ability to properly absorb nutrients. Asparagus spears can be eaten raw, and just four spears per day will give you all the benefits to be had from this essential superfood.

Brussels sprouts

You may have always heard that you should eat your Brussels sprouts, but if you've ignored this then you have been depriving your body of some amazing benefits. Consistently rated as one of the top superfoods, Brussels sprouts are bursting at the seams with essential vitamins such as C and K. If it's fiber you're after, you can certainly find it here as well.

One of the main benefits of Brussels sprouts is their lowering of cholesterol. When consumed regularly, these beneficial sprouts can even significantly eliminate harmful cholesterol. All you need is one sprout per serving and there are many delicious ways to prepare them. As a side dish to a main meal, Brussels sprouts will have you well on your way to a healthier diet.

Kale

When it comes to vitamins, there is a reason that kale consistently sits at the top of the superfoods list. You won't find many other foods this high in essential vitamins. The main vitamin trio in kale is A, C, and K. Vitamin A helps out with bone growth and strength, boosts the immune system, and even aids in reproduction. Vitamin C is effective as a powerful antioxidant that cleans out the system, and vitamin K regulates bone loss and helps the body bounce back quickly from injuries. At only 8 calories per cup serving, Kale is truly an essential superfood that no healthy diet should be without.

Collard Greens

Similar to kale, collard greens are jam packed with the essential vitamins your body needs to perform a wide variety of beneficial internal operations. The vitamin A in this vegetable will aid in bone growth, the health of your immune system, and in reproductive functions. The vitamin C will bring into play all its beneficial antioxidant qualities, and the vitamin K will help to assist your body's immune system functioning. Additionally, collard greens have cholesterol lowering functions that can be life savers down the line. As a vegetable that offers both vitamin goodness and cholesterol-lowering ability, collard greens truly deserve their place in the superfoods spectrum. For any superfood diet, a regular cup serving of kale should certainly be worked into the routine.

Ladies' Fingers

These refreshing pods have everything you need when it comes to a superfood. Not only are they an incredibly rich source of vitamins C and K but they are also full of essential minerals and fiber. As an added bonus, ladies' fingers contain iron, calcium, and manganese. This puts these attractive pods firmly at the top of the superfoods list. You just won't find a food more packed with goodness. Just 8 of these tiny pods in a serving will get you started right, and they taste great so that should never be a problem.

Leafy Greens: Spinach and Swiss Chard

Leafy greens like spinach and Swiss chard are jam packed with nutrients. There are a plethora of nutrients including vitamins A, B, C, E, and K, as well as fiber, copper, calcium, zinc, magnesium and so much more. These aid in cardiovascular protection, energy fortification, immune system building, boosts brain function, amplifies night vision, and stabilizes blood sugar. Because there are so many nutrients you just can't go wrong adding these to your diet. Hint: They are wonderful in smoothies and I promise you won't even know they are in there!

Avocados

Avocados are nutrient dense fruit and are actually one berry but with only a single seed. By eating an avocado, you receive 1/3 of your daily requirement for vitamin K, Vitamin B6, vitamin C, pantothenic acid, folate, and much more.

While bananas are great, avocados have twice the potassium. Avocados have glutathione, which aids in preventing many types of cancers and kill the pre-cancerous cells that are involved with the formation of cancer. They are also an extremely healthy fat.

Chia seeds

Much like the rest of the super foods on this list, chia seeds also give an immense amount of nutrients. The root word, chia, stands for "strength" in an ancient Mayan language. Since the growth of fitness and health on social media outlets like Instagram, chia seeds have been bursting in popularity. A single ounce of the very small seeds only has 137 calories and only 1g of carbohydrate. Without the protein in the chia seeds, they would only be 101 calories. Crazy!

Walnuts

Also known as the super food nut, walnuts have omega-3 fatty acids including alpha linolenic acid, canola oil, flaxseed and the oil derived from such, spinach, purslane, and even plant sterols. This aids in helping decrease cholesterol levels. They also provide protein, copper, magnesium, folate and vitamin e. A normal serving is a fourth of a cup and is only up to 200 calories.

Broccoli

Broccoli is a super food rich in fiber, and antioxidants to ward off cancer and prevent other ailments. There is also vitamin C to help those who need to benefit from iron absorption.

There's also beta-carotene, vitamins A and K, calcium, fiber, and much more packed into this green.

Simple, Healthy, and Positive

When consuming a toxic diet you are filling your body with pollutants that drain your energy, cloud your thoughts, and keep your body from performing at the level it deserves. Consuming superfoods will not only boost your bodily health but will significantly aid positive thinking and overall mood.

You deserve a healthy body, positive mind power, and an improved outlook on life. Superfoods will give you all of this and much more.

As you can see from the list, superfoods are not hard to track down, complicated to consume, or overly expensive. These are simple plant-based foods that can be found in any supermarket, specialty store, or fruit and vegetable cart. All that you have to do is start incorporating these foods into your diet while phasing out the toxic foods that you've been consuming.

Once you start to feel the benefits of these superfoods it will be easier to resist the cravings for junk foods and fast foods since you know they are doing you harm while the superfoods are doing your body and mind right. Before you know it you will be on a superfood diet and benefiting fully from all of the nutrients and benefits these foods bring to the table.

Now that you understand the benefits of superfoods, the negatives of a toxic diet, and have your list of the top simple and healthy superfoods that will greatly benefit your body and mind, the time is right to make a change today.

Get rid of that toxic diet that is doing you harm and treat yourself to a healthy and positive diet of superfoods that pack the vitamins, minerals, and other beneficial ingredients your body has been craving. Once you have begun experiencing benefits such as increased energy, better mood, glowing skin, and positive mental outlook, you won't miss the toxic diet you have left behind. Start up your superfood diet today and truly unlock your better self.

How to Get Started With a Liver Detox

All liver detox programs advocate the purging of harmful toxins from the liver. The challenge is finding which program you should follow. While it can be confusing to choose one detox program over another, what really matters is that you choose one that helps you cleanse your liver without any dangerous side-effects or drastic methods.

For example, some programs may promote the benefits of an all liquid diet for a period of several days or even weeks. This is not a realistic or healthy approach to any diet plan, especially one that is supposed to heal your body.

One of the best approaches is a liver cleanse that is based on superfoods that specifically detox the body and support healthy liver function. You eat nothing but whole, nutrient dense foods that will reboot and rejuvenate your body – all without starving yourself or taking drastic measures like a liquid fast.

How long should you stay on a liver cleanse program? Optimally, a period of about 10 -14 days is best so that it gives your body time to acclimate to the new food plan and work its magic to heal you from head to toe.

However, if you live a very busy lifestyle and feel that a full liver detox is difficult to follow, then you can try this alternate version.

What you do is eat a cup of raw grated beets mixed with lemon juice and olive oil for 30 days.

You eat this mixture before breakfast. You also need to drink liver detox tea at least once a day.

(**NOTE**: It is much easier, and more effective, to perform a 10-day full liver detox than choosing the 30-day alternative just discussed. As you probably know, it is easier to adhere to 10 days of behavioral changes than it is to religiously go 30 full days following any type of procedure. The choice is yours, but you will probably find the 10-day full liver detox delivers quicker results and is easier to stick to because it is much shorter in length. You will also see the rewards of your efforts much sooner and this provides a lot of motivation to keep going.)

What to Expect with a Liver Detox?

The full liver detox removes gallstones that might have formed in the gallbladder, as well as other toxins, poisons and other harmful substances you have ingested.

Your liver detox may also be accompanied by symptoms such as fatigue, body odor, nausea, headache, body aches and insomnia. **This is the body's normal reaction to the detoxification process. Those symptoms are a wonderful sign you are becoming healthier!**

The toxins the liver has removed are transported to the gastrointestinal tract for waste disposal. Some of these toxins might leak into the blood stream, causing discomfort. It is normal for the body to react negatively as the reaction is similar to withdrawal from alcohol or drugs by an addict.

Your body is cleansing yourself of poisons which you and may have spent years eating and drinking.

Removing them from your body in a relatively short period of time is sometimes hard for your body to take.

Don't be alarmed. Your liver, and the rest of your body, is returning to its healthy natural state. After your liver detox is done, you will feel energetic and vibrant, you will experience healthy weight loss, you will find your thinking clear and sharp, and you will enjoy all the wonderful health benefits mentioned earlier.

Sample Liver Detox Plan

Now it is time to actually put your knowledge to practice. You should be getting excited, because in a very short period of time, you will begin to look and feel better than you have in years, possibly even decades. Get started today, follow this sample detox plan, and weight loss, "all day" energy, healthy, young, strong looking and feeling skin and hair and a sharper mind will be your rewards.

Relying on the right foods during your liver detox plan is very important as it can aid your liver to get rid of more toxins. While there are many who swear by the efficacy of juicing to cleanse their liver, this is sometimes hard to maintain, especially in the long run. *It is extremely important that you strictly follow the liver detox plan but it is also important that you eat the right foods to create optimal liver health.* This chapter discusses what you need to know about eating for a healthy liver.

Tips for a Healthy Liver Diet

Once you learn what to eat, you can ensure your liver continues to function at a healthy level for the rest of your life. It is important you choose the right foods to avoid complicating the conditions of a toxic liver. The right foods will help you hasten the speed of your cleanse as you feed your body foods that will not overwork your liver.

Upon waking drink a glass of hot lemon water. This is an essential part of any liver detox program. It helps to flush the liver of toxins and alkalizes the body.

Squeeze the juice from ½ a lemon into 8 ounces of hot or warm water.

Eat foods that have low salt: Remember that too much salt can overwork your kidneys and this organ is essential for successful liver detox. Both kidneys and liver work hand and hand to properly cleanse your body of waste.

Eat foods that are low in fat: High fatty foods can endanger your liver as they can overwork your organ to produce more bile to break down fats. The exception here is healthy fats like those found in avocados and coconut oil. However, even these foods should be limited.

More fiber: Fiber helps the liver slow down its absorption of glucose. This helps you regulate a healthy body weight. Remember that glucose is stored in the liver and the faster it is transported to the liver, the higher chances of developing fatty liver disease. The presence of fiber from fruits and vegetables slows down the uptake of glucose by the liver.

Avoid fast foods and processed foods: This one is self-explanatory. Fast food items and processed foods, foods which come in a wrapper, container, box or can, contain high amounts of fats, salt, trans fats, MSG (monosodium glutamate) and sugar which, impede the proper functioning of the liver. Those unhealthy food items also cause a long list of other health problems. This includes, but is certainly not limited to, snacks, pastries, baked goods, candies, fried foods and soda drinks.

Avoid alcohol of all kinds. Alcohol does nothing good for your liver or the rest of your body. It causes your liver to work overtime to break it down and rid the body of it. If you have gotten into the habit of having a "night cap" to help you sleep, take this time to break it.

Alcohol does not help to promote restful sleep. In fact, it does the complete opposite – it damages your sleep cycle. Among other negative consequences, poor sleep will further impact your liver because it is during sleep that the liver really does its job of cleansing your body. Bottom line – stay away from it.

Menu Suggestions

Food preparation for a healthy liver detox need not be complicated. Below are some simple meal suggestions that you can prepare to achieve a healthy liver cleanse.

Breakfast:

Eat oats or whole grain bread with skim milk. Other breakfast options include a piece of banana and fresh fruit juice or yogurt mixed with berries. You can also drink black coffee as research suggests that black coffee is very beneficial to the liver. (Limit your coffee consumption to no more than 2 small cups, and skip the cream and sugar.)

Lunch:

Avoid cheese and red meat. Go for white meats like chicken or turkey. Eat organic whenever you can. You can also consume vegetable soup or a clear consommé and a tossed salad. Do not consume sweet desserts like cake or other types of decadent pastries. Instead, opt for fruits.

Make sure to drink lemon water to wash down your meals.

Snacks:

Snacks can be any type of salt-free nuts, celery, carrot sticks or dark chocolate. (Keep your dark chocolate consumption confined to natural, organic products with no added sugar and other harmful ingredients.) You can also eat plums, raisins or any fruit of your choice.

Dinner:

You can eat a large dinner but do not eat beyond the capacity of your stomach. Give yourself time to process the food that you eat, chewing thoroughly. If you listen to your body, it will tell you when you are full. Choose white meat or fish, insisting upon wild caught fish as opposed to farm raised.

If you opt for chicken, make sure that you do not fry it. Add any type of vegetable dishes that are steamed, roasted or baked. Drink lemon water or skim milk to finish your meals.

Below is an example of a one-day diet plan for a healthy liver detox.

Breakfast:

- 4 slices of fruit

- Lemon Water

Lunch:

- Vegetable Salad

- 1 roasted Rainbow trout

- 3 pieces of artichoke hearts

- ½ tbsp. toasted sesame seeds

Snacks:

- 2 plums

- 6 almonds

Dinner:

- 1/3 cup cooked brown rice

- 1 cup of boiled lentils

- ½ cup sautéed mushrooms

- Large vegetable salad

- Lemon juice

When preparing healthy liver detox meals, you can vary them so that you are comfortable with the food you eat. It is important to take note that you don't have to sacrifice your enjoyment to food while you are doing a liver detox. ***What is important is you choose your food wisely.***

Detox Infographic

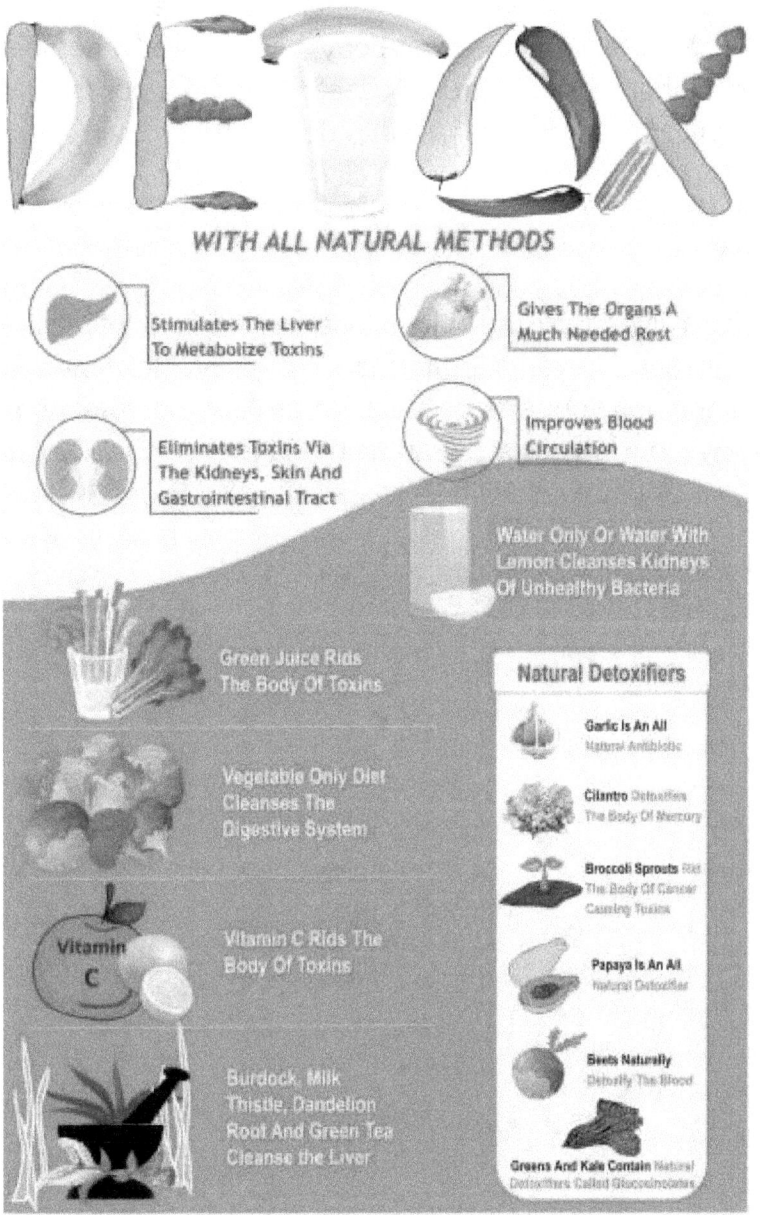

Conclusion

When your liver is unhealthy, your body becomes toxic. When contaminants and toxins are not removed from your body, this leads to a number of health conditions. In extreme cases, ignoring a poorly functioning liver can even lead to death.

Fortunately, the answer is simple – *a healthy, natural liver detox.*

A natural liver detox helps you lose weight, fight infection and disease, prevents the formation of painful liver stones and improves your energy level. You return a natural and healthy glow to your skin and hair, and look and feel younger with a liver detox as well.

Other Senior Health and Fitness Books by This Author

If you would like to read more about Senior Health and Fitness, here is a list of the titles, CreateSpace links and descriptions:

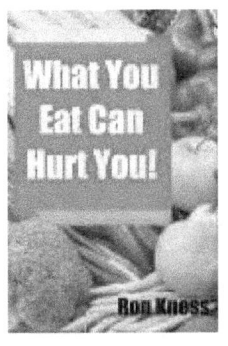

What You Eat Can Hurt You

https://www.createspace.com/4963196

Do you know that certain foods increase your risk for inflammation, disease and illness? It's true! And certain foods can help cure and heal you if you do get sick. Knowing which foods to eat and which ones to avoid empowers you to manage your own health.

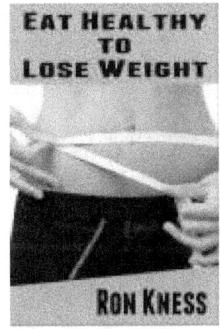

Eat Healthy to Lose Weight

https://www.createspace.com/4962939

As you read through our book, we show you which foods you should and should not be eating to reach your weight loss goal, along with discussing how to maintain your weight loss and stay within a few pounds of your goal weight. Banish the weight you keep gaining back each time by learning how to live a healthy lifestyle.

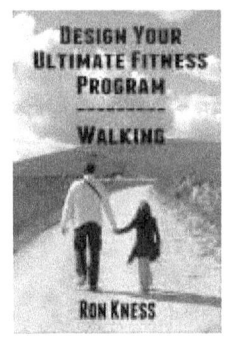 Design Your Ultimate Fitness Program - Walking

https://www.createspace.com/5252272

In my book Design Your Ultimate Fitness Program – Walking, we discuss the considerations that need to be made when designing a custom walking program, along with:

• Equipment needed
• Wearable technology you can use to track your walking
• And how to make walking more challenging

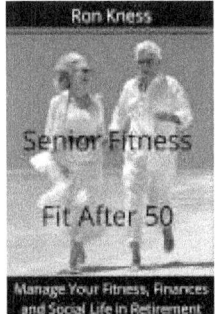 Senior Fitness – Fit After 50: Learn How to Manage Your Fitness, Finances and Social Life in Retirement

https://www.createspace.com/5474751

Inside you will discover answers to your most pressing questions:
• What do I need to know about downsizing my home?
• What are the best tips for staying healthy as you approach your 50's?
• When should I start planning for retirement?
• I am worried about being lonely once I retire, do others feel the same?
• Is it worthwhile to carry two homes during retirement?
And more…

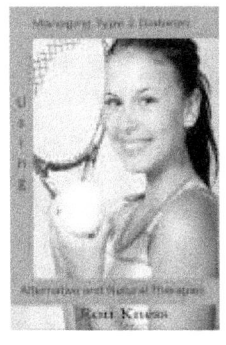

Managing Type 2 Diabetes Using Alternative And Natural Therapies

https://www.createspace.com/5401244

While Type 2 diabetes can be managed medically, there are many alternative natural and holistic methods of therapy and treatment that can further enhance quality of life and minimize the effects of this disease. In this book, I discuss 12 different types, including yoga, reflexology and acupuncture to name just three.

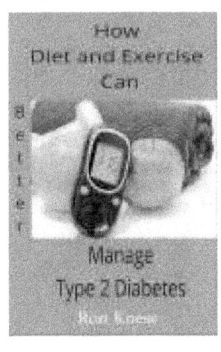

How Diet and Exercise Can Better Manage Type 2 Diabetes

https://www.createspace.com/5404845

Of the different types of diabetes, only Type 2 can be reversed. In my book How Diet and Exercise Can Better Manage Type 2 Diabetes, we reveal the three things you can do to best manage your disease, including:
• Diet
• Exercise
• Weight management

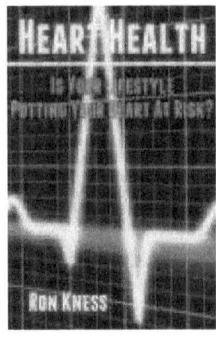

Heart Health: Is Your Lifestyle Putting Your Heart at Risk?

https://www.createspace.com/5464020

In my ebook Is Your Lifestyle Putting Your Heart At Risk? we discuss the six greatest risks to your heart and the lifestyle changes you can make to mitigate them.

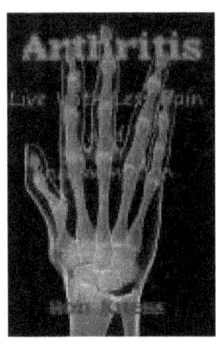

Arthritis – Live Wth Less Pain and Inflammation: Tips and Techniques You Can Use to Lessen the Pain and Inflammation

https://www.createspace.com/5457441

Discover Simple Tips & Information That Will Help Reduce The Painful Symptoms Of Arthritis!

You learn things like:
• Simple and effective information that will help you manage the pain and inflammation that comes along with arthritis, so that you can live an active, full life without debilitating pain.
• The different types of arthritis, their symptoms and how to alleviate their painful side effects.
• The pros and cons of over-the-counter arthritis medications, plus simple tips that will help you know how to choose the right supplements.
• Free, yet effective ways to get relief from arthritis pain and inflammation, so you don't have to suffer anymore.

the effects arthritis can have significant impact on your physical and mental well-being, but this books shows you how to overcome its painful symptoms and live life relatively pain free.

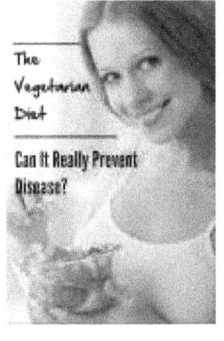

The Vegetarian Diet – Can It Really Prevent Disease?

https://www.createspace.com/5519874

Is a vegetarian diet right for you? Multiple studies have shown over and over that a vegetarian diet goes along way in preventing certain chronic diseases, such as:

- Heart Disease
- Cancer
- Diverticulitis
- Type 2 Diabetes
- Hypertension
- Obesity
- Kidney Failure

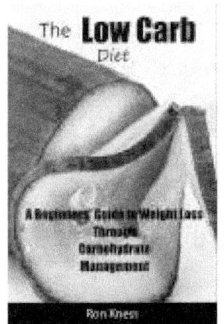

The Low Carb Diet: A Beginner's Guide to Weight Loss Through Carbohydrate Management

https://www.createspace.com/5416348

In my book "The Low-Carb Diet – A Beginners' Guide to Weight Loss Through Carbohydrate Management", I reveal a successful method of losing weight based in part on the amount and type of carbohydrates you consume.

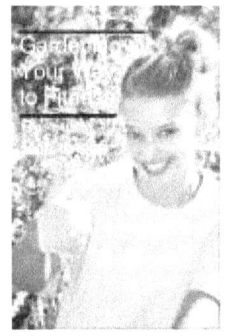

Gardening Your Way to Fitness: The Fun Way to Get Fit and Provide Beauty and Healthful Bounty for Your Family

https://www.createspace.com/5459564

The gym is a great place to stay fit during the colder seasons, but once the temperature turns warmer you want to spend more time outside. Plus, you'll have the benefit of fresh wholesome produce to enjoy by growing vegetables in your backyard garden.

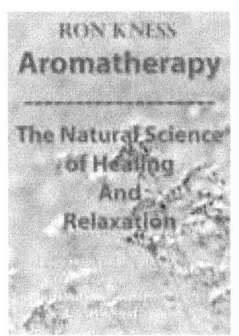

Aromatherapy - The Science of Healing and Relaxation: Learn How Essential Oils Elicit The Relaxation Response And Alter Mood

https://www.createspace.com/5714434

In my book Aromatherapy – The Science of Healing and Relaxation, we reveal the natural holistics methods you can use to heal the body from certain medical issues and to relive stress through relaxation. In particular we talk about:
• Aromatherapy - what it is and how it works
• Essential Oils – how the effects of certain aromas differs from others
• Recipes – how to make your own essential oil combinations

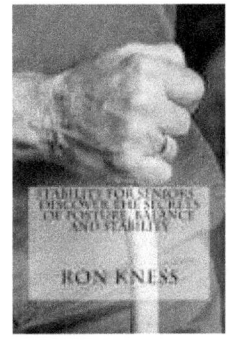

<u>Stability for Seniors</u>: <u>Discover the Secrets of Posture, Balance and Stability</u>

https://www.createspace.com/6096479

Many people sacrifice their health in pursuit of their career. They are so busy making a living that they neglect to make a life. The excuse that they do not have time to exercise is tossed about so frequently that they end up letting their health and fitness slide.

If you are not regularly active, you will have muscular atrophy over time. Your flexibility will decrease. Your core strength will diminish. As time progresses, you will be less limber and more rigid.

This is exactly how people age poorly. It's a process that has snowballed over time.

Only with regular exercise and a healthy diet can you have a body that is fit and has the ability to almost reverse aging.

If you have neglected your health for years and life seems to be a chore now because you can't get around without assistance, do not feel dejected.

You can remedy the situation. You can restore the strength, balance and stamina that you have lost. It is never too late to become what you might have been.

This guide will show you exactly what you need to do to restore your balance, strengthen your core and give you the ability to live life to its fullest. Read how …

About the Author

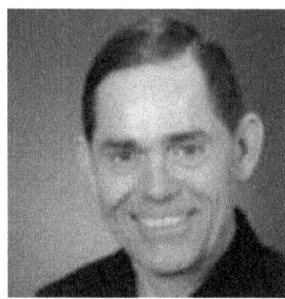

I grew up in Central Minnesota, where my parents owned and operated a fishing resort. Once out of high school I tried a couple of semesters of college, only to quit halfway through the Spring term; I decided at that time that college wasn't for me.

Then I decided to follow my father's previous occupation as an auto mechanic. I graduated from a two-year of vocational training course and worked as a mechanic. While in vocational training, I decided to join the National Guard where I eventually ended up working full-time for 32 years.

So how does all of this relate to writing? In one of my leadership schools, the instructor, who was an English teacher at a juvenile detention center, presented writing to me in a whole new way - a way that started to develop my interest in working with words.

Fast forward about 40 years and I now have over 50 books listed on Amazon for Kindle and CreateSpace.

Besides my own writing, I also ghostwrite ebooks, reports, articles, blogs and do Kindle conversions for my clients on a variety of topics.

Today my wife and I live in Gold Canyon, AZ, where you'll find me happily sitting in my office typing away on my laptop as I work on my next book or ghostwriting project . . . that is if we are not traveling on a cruise ship - our new-found mode of travel.

www.ingramcontent.com/pod-product-compliance
Lightning Source LLC
Chambersburg PA
CBHW060647290526
45793CB00001B/440